# The Power of Plants

## Why You Should Eat More

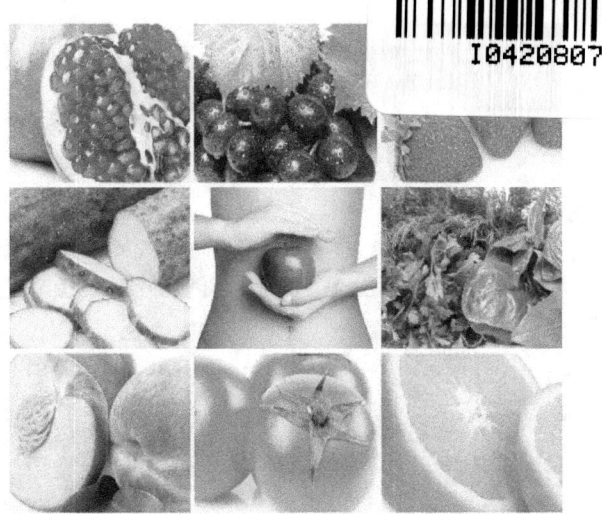

By

## Michael K

leahciM K

storage of this document is not allowed unless with written permission from the publisher. All rights reserved.

The information provided herein is stated to be truthful and consistent, in that any liability, in terms of inattention or otherwise, by any usage or abuse of any policies, processes, or directions contained within is the solitary and utter responsibility of the recipient reader. Under no circumstances will any legal responsibility or blame be held against the publisher for any reparation, damages, or monetary loss due to the information herein, either directly or indirectly.

Respective authors own all copyrights not held by the publisher.

The information herein is offered for informational purposes solely, and is universal as so. The presentation of the information is without contract or any type of guarantee assurance.

leahciM K

.

# Table of Contents

# INTRODUCTION

If you wish to be more friendly to the global environment, economy, and also your own body and mind — cut back on meat, dairy, other animal products, and processed foods. It really is that simple, but no one expects you to make any big changes without first learning more about the topic. This book has been carefully created by someone who is passionate about the benefits of eating more plant-based foods, and cutting down on the amount of animal-based products consumed.

There seems to be a global conspiracy *against* eating plants. For quite some time, the popular believe has been that eating food from animals is more natural.

With so much information indicating the exact opposite these days, it's a wonder that such a high number of the population still clings to this archaic and *unnatural* point of view.

If you take a look at the way the media has portrayed vegetarians and vegans over the past decades, it starts to become apparent just *why* people think this way. Everyone seems to have been brainwashed by people who don't care a lot about public health and wellbeing. The meat and dairy industries don't care whether you live a long, healthy life, or if you have a heart attack at the age of 50. Do you think they are actually doing research to try and give people accurate information about their products? It's far more likely that they are just trying to come up with information that helps them make money. Yes, you could say the same about the industries that sell vegetables, fruits, etc. The choice is really your own to make, in the end. Should you read through this book, and decide that the information presented within it are a load of garbage — that's fine. But please, do give it a chance, and consider adopting at least some of the core ideas into your own life.

# Top Myths About Meat-Free Diets

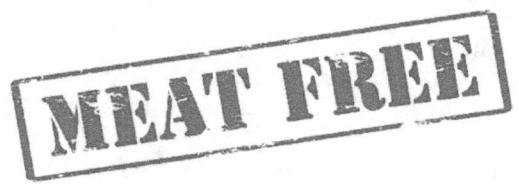

There's a lot of *smack* being talked about plant-based diets, especially as they become more popular in the media, among celebrities, and public figures. Please, do your own research and decide for yourself. Just realize that there is a lot of heat around the topic, with people getting all worked up, while ignoring many facts. Here are some of the most common myths that you are sure to come across:

### *"You need to eat meat for protein"*

Protein is a big thing at the moment, and it seems that everyone wants to shovel down chicken and beef in order to get more than enough. Meat is not the only way to get protein, and it can actually come from most different types of foods. An ounce of meat has around the same protein as half a cup of beans, so this myth is blatantly false.

### *"You can't bulk up as a vegan"*

You don't need to eat meat or animal products to be a top athlete, as many people have already proved. You can certainly give your body plenty of fuel for exercise, with a completely plant-based diet. It might take more thought that just eating lots of steak and eggs (which isn't such a great idea anyway), but you can get great results, all the same.

### *"Vegan food is gross"*

This seems like something a child might think, but there are lots of adults who still hate the idea of eating their veggies. If you have the mindset that you'll be eating nothing but salads, it's bound to sound pretty boring. It's important to experiment, and start to learn about all the great types of foods that can be enjoyed, with no meat. It will take some time for most people's taste buds to adapt to a new diet, but just stick with it until that happens.

### *"Vegan diets cause definite weight loss"*

There are lots of vegans and vegetarians who are overweight, although probably more of the latter than the former. People can still eat a lot of junk food, even without eating any meat or other animal products. No matter what type of foods you eat, losing weight takes careful planning and effort.

**"Meat is essential for pregnancy"**

You probably shouldn't choose to mess around with your existing diet, while pregnant. However, if a woman is already vegan or vegetarian, and following a healthy eating plan — there is no reason why she should start to eat meat after becoming pregnant. This is a discussion that's best had with your doctor, however.

*"Meat-free food costs too much"*

Yes, wholesome and nutritious food does cost more than junk food. If you want to compare a healthy, plant-based diet with a diet of processed foods, you're going to get the skewed view of things. Meat is one of the most expensive things that you can buy, and there's no avoiding that. You should actually start to save money on a plant-based diet. Fresh fruits and vegetables are typically less than even the cheaper cuts of meat, and whole grains are often affordable.

### *"You'll always be tired"*

If you switch to a plant-based diet, full of whole foods, you should be anything *but* tired. Often, people find that they feel more energetic when they cut meat and animal foods from their diets. If you do find that your energy levels feel depleted, there's a good chance that you're missing out on something important. Lowered levels of iron and B12 are commonly a problem for new vegans and vegetarians. You need to be sure that you're eating foods like legumes and spinach, which contain lots of iron. As for B12, you'll need to get that from a supplement, or from dairy and eggs.

### "You need to starve yourself"

Just take a look at some of the different foods listed in this book. Do you think that you would go hungry eating them? If you do go meat-free, and you're feeling hungry all the time, something isn't right. All of the fiber that's found in plant-based foods helps to keep your stomach fuller for longer, so you might need to closely look at what you're eating. Maybe something important is being left out, which should be rectified as quickly as possible.

### *"You're all in, or all out"*

You don't have to go totally vegan to get the benefits of eating more vegan foods. Just cutting down the amount of meat, dairy, and eggs that you consume, can reduce your chances of developing heart disease, cancer, and diabetes, to name just a few things. Even if you only remove one or two servings of meat from your weekly diet, it will have results. There's no need to go "overboard" and make your life unsatisfying. If you really do love meat that much, just try not to eat it too often. Like all things in life, the art here is to find a good balance.

### *"You need to eat faux-meat"*

There are lots of fake "meat" products out there. Most meat eaters probably assume that these are a staple of vegan diets. However, many people choose to eat other foods instead. Meat substitutes are often not very healthy, since they are loaded with additives and preservatives. In many cases, it might be healthier to just eat real meat instead.

# Key Benefits of Eating More Plants

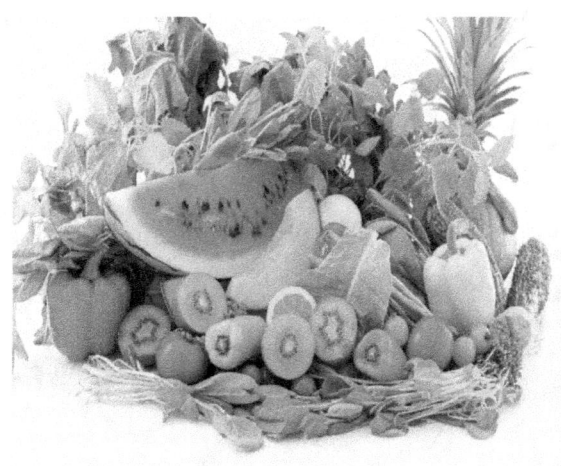

After introducing more plants into their diets, or actually going 100% vegan, people generally notice some wonderful benefits. Please, be assured that this is certainly not a coincidence. The feeling of wellbeing that comes with cutting down on animal products, and introducing lots of whole foods, also comes with many other health benefits.

Animal foods are typically processed a lot more than food that comes from plants, but that's just one small part of the problem. Since animals are living, breathing creatures, with mental and physical feelings, it doesn't make sense to use them in such a barbaric way. Not only does it cost *loads* of money, but it works to gradually destroy the environment as well. In the end, the outcome is a whole host of health problems for people who eat meat and other animal products. Does that sound like a good trade to you? Who really wins when the human population of earth decides to eat steak, bacon, eggs, or dairy, instead of fresh fruits, vegetables, and cereals? It doesn't seem like there are any real winners, apart from the people who are profiting from the meat and dairy industries.

## *Health*

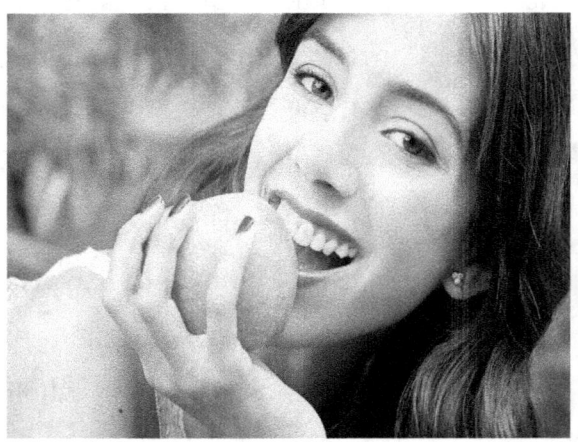

You might have heard people claiming that animal-based foods are bad for humans, but probably still want to see some specific information. Here are some of the major health benefits that come from eating a primarily, or entirely, plant-based diet. Eating lots of plants can help you to stay healthy, or even recover from poor health. The scientific evidence is overwhelming at this point in time. It shows that a diet based around whole plant-based foods, can combat a huge range of diseases, including diabetes, heart disease, inflammation, osteoporosis, cancer, and many more.

## *Cholesterol*

This is a key benefit that comes with starting a plant-based diet. Instead of worrying about just how much your next meal or snack will clog up your arteries, enjoy something that is cholesterol free. Many people do not realize that plants don't have any cholesterol in them, even if they are higher in saturated fats, as with cacao and coconut. While it's still important to balance how much fat you consume, vegans don't often have to worry about their cholesterol. Many vegan foods actually work to lower the amount of cholesterol that's in the body, and combat heart disease. Even if you don't plan to stop eating meat and other animal-based foods, cutting down is a great way to take care of a nasty cholesterol problem.

## *Cancer*

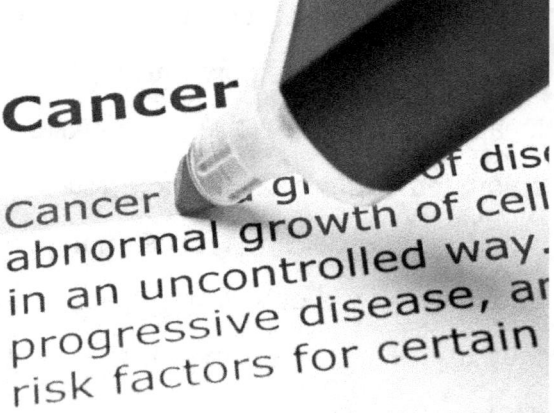

Like most people, the thought of cancer probably terrifies you. There are a lot of things that supposedly cause, or contribute to, the growth of cancers. While scientists are still learning a lot about it, there is some great news for people who want healthy ways to limit their chances of developing it. You can do this by using the power of plants!

Cancer is known to begin in the damaged cells of the body. In order to prevent this from happening, it is essential to work to keep your body's cells in top condition. There is a lot of research that indicates that whole vegetables and fruits can help to protect against harm to cells in the body.

A comprehensive analysis, released in the *Annals of Nutrition & Metabolism* medical review, took into account a number of studies. These were some of the best studies that have been undertaken, with information about mortality rates and causes. It shows that vegetarians can expect a largely lower rate of cancer. While vegetarians still eat animal products, cutting meat out of their diet clearly lead to a healthier lifestyle. (You can see this analysis for yourself here: www.karger.com/Article/Pdf/337301.)

If vegetarians are less likely to develop cancer, what about vegans? A study was funded by the National Cancer Institute, and released by the Loma Linda University. It shows that vegans are less likely to get cancer, than vegetarians or people who eat meat. (Here is a link to that study: www.ncbi.nlm.nih.gov/pubmed/2316992

9.)

Research that was published in the *Cell Metabolism* journal, showed that middle aged people who had diets with lots of animal protein, had a quadrupled chance of dying from cancer. The researchers observed the health and diets of over 6,000 people, over the age of 50, over a period of 18 years. The information was taken from a national dietary survey in the United States. While this research showed that high levels of protein were linked to cancer, it also showed that this problem almost entirely went away — when the protein came from plants instead.

No one expects you to become an expert in the science behind all of this. However, it is important to make sure the evidence is there, before you adopt any type of new diet for good health. For a long time, many people have mocked plant eaters, claiming that they are both unhealthy, and foolish. It is very encouraging to see that the scientific research is strongly backing up vegans and vegetarians at last.

## *Blood Sugar Levels*

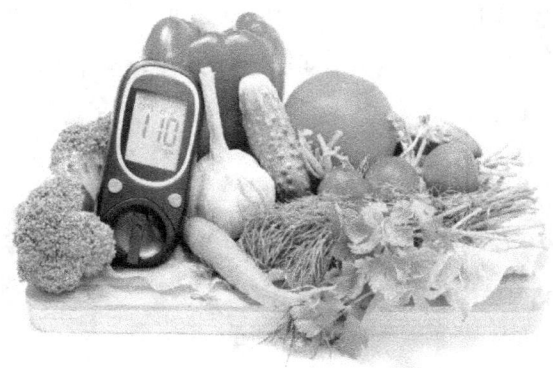

Eating lots of fiber is important for fighting against high blood sugar. And what is one of the best ways to get more fiber into your diet? No, there's no need to start taking any expensive supplements, because fruits, vegetables, and cereals contain *loads* of natural fiber. Since fiber can slow down the speed at which the blood stream absorbs sugars, it can leave you feeling fuller for longer, while keeping cortisol levels balanced.

## Digestive System

Have you ever had troubles with keeping bowel movements regular? Constipation is a common problem, especially with so many people failing to eat healthy diets, and drink enough water. There are millions of dollars spent on supplements, pharmaceuticals, herbal treatments, vitamins, and laxatives — all in order to do something that is meant to come naturally. This can be fixed by some pretty simple dietary changes. Eating lots of good plants can rapidly get rid of constipation, without the need to take anything else.

## *Lower Blood Pressure*

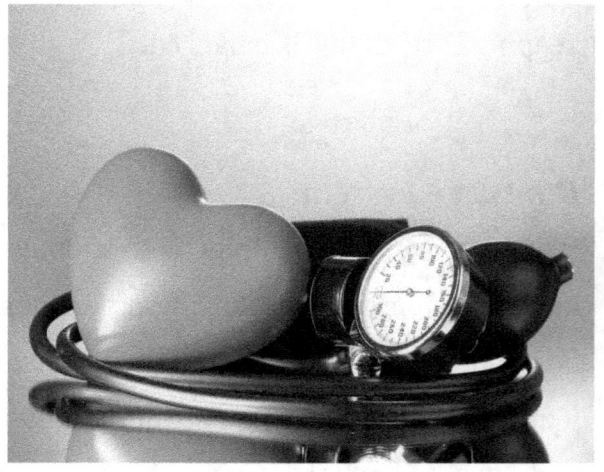

People who eat diets filled mainly with plants, simply have lower blood pressure, on average. This is largely because they are eating such a great range of foods that are high in potassium, among other things. Potassium is known to reduce blood pressure, which can also reduce anxiety and stress. Instead of eating meat for protein and other things, vegans and vegetarians turn to legumes, grains, seeds, nuts, fruits, and vegetables, to meet their dietary needs. These foods are wonderfully rich in Vitamin B6 too, which is another substance known to lower blood pressure.

## *Weight Loss*

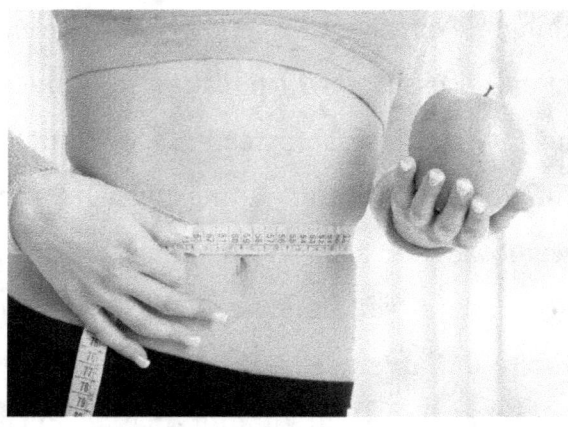

Many people reading this book have probably decided to look into a plant-based diet for one big reason — to lose weight. While there are loads of other reasons to stop eating so many animal products, weight loss is certainly one of the most appealing. Can you really shed those unwanted pounds, and keep them gone, by making some relatively simple dietary changes? Don't you need to starve yourself and give up ever feeling full? Are there a whole bunch of crazy and expensive recipes that a person needs to eat, to stick to a healthy and slimming vegan diet? The answer to these questions is an emphatic "no".

# Why Do Vegan Diets Work?

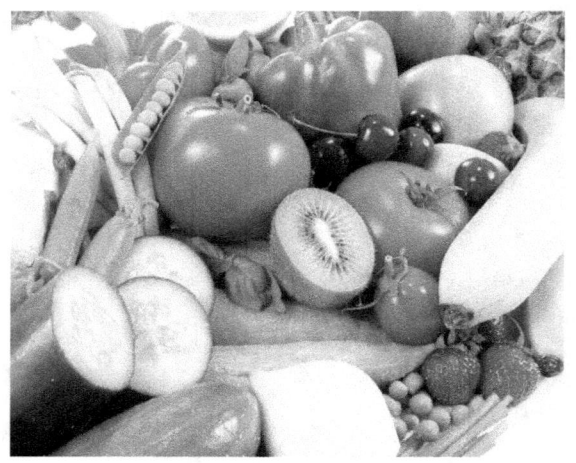

When someone becomes a vegan, they will generally start to lose some weight. You might believe that this is due to being "malnourished". That's certainly what pro-active meat lovers will tell you, anyway. The truth is, people tend to lose weight because they are introducing *much* more fiber into their diets. Eating foods with lots of fiber helps to cleanse your insides, pushing out a whole lot of junk from the intestinal system. This is why eating more plants can help to alleviate constipation, as mentioned in this chapter.

If you provide your body with enough fiber every day, you will continually be cleaning out your intestines. Take a look at food that comes from animals instead. It doesn't have fiber at all! This includes all of those so called "healthy" and "necessary" foods like, beef, lamb, pork, chicken, turkey, fish, cheese, eggs, and milk. That's right, you will not get your daily dose of fiber from these things, but they do have a whole lot of calories, fats, etc.

If you were to go to the gym and have a trainer give you some advice, they might say to eat more chicken, fish, and other "healthy" animal products. Lean meats are typically viewed as healthy options for weight loss and exercise routines. You can lose weight with a more traditional diet, and you might get rid of some other health problems for some time. Eventually, there's a big chance that the weight is going to come back. With a vegan diet, or even a vegetarian diet that's low on animal products — you can lose weight and actually keep it gone.

## *Great Tips for Vegan Weight Loss*

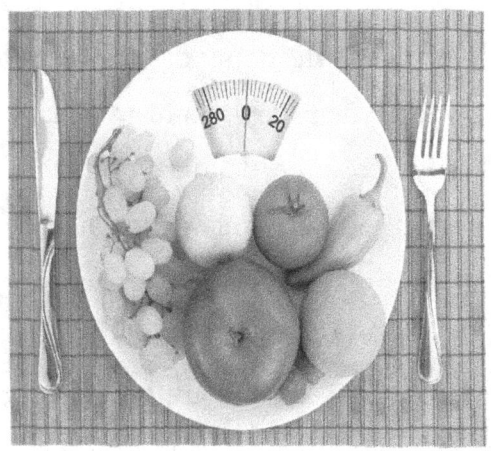

Starting a vegan diet can be pretty tough, so you will need some help. These tips are designed to give you some quick guidance, so that you don't make any major mistakes in the beginning of your new dietary journey.

1. If you look at the recommended foods that vegans should eat, it might seem like a lot. Those guidelines are intended for

people who are at a healthy weight already, or even looking to gain a little weight. This all depends on just how much you weigh now, your gender, and a whole host of other factors. Don't assume that eating vegan food will automatically cause you to lose weight. It's necessary to monitor how *much* you are consuming as well. To lose weight, you need to eat less calories than you are burning up with daily activities and exercise. That means it's probably necessary to eat *less* than the recommended amount. Of course, this book is not intended as a thorough guide to weight loss. It's best to ask your doctor, and find some other resources that are dedicated to losing weight. Just don't let anyone tell you that a vegan diet is anything but great.

2. Eat more whole grains, because they are wonderfully for overall health, as well as losing weight. White flour, pasta, and other grains, simply have much of the natural goodness removed. This includes a lot of the fiber, which is necessary for health, so eating refined grains is a bad idea. Whole grains are a wonderful source of complex carbohydrates too. However, you should not go overboard on how much you eat, especially while trying to slim down.

3. Don't replace meat or dairy with "faux" products. There are lots of vegan alternatives on the supermarket shelves, such as soy cheeses and meats. These are fine to enjoy occasionally, but they are usually far from being healthy. They are often high in salt and fat. Once you reach

your desired weight, it is okay to eat more of these pre-packaged foods, in moderation.

4. Be careful about sugar intake, even if it is in the form of vegan foods. It can be easy to fall into the "healthy" sugar trap. Even fruits contain high amounts of sugar, generally, so you have to limit how many you eat. Just because a smoothie contains lots of fruits, it doesn't automatically make it healthy. Fruit juices are also a big culprit here, so it's best to avoid them entirely. Once again, this is linked largely to the fiber that's missing from juiced fruits. You're better off blending your fruits and vegetables, so that you can get *all* of the goodness, instead of concentrated sugar and acids.

5. Drink water, drink water, and *drink water*. If you start to eat more fiber-rich foods, you're going to need to drink enough water. Otherwise, you will run the risk of becoming constipated for a whole different reason. A ballpark amount of water to aim for each day is 6 to 12 glasses per day, of eight ounces each. This varies from person to person, and also depends on what you are eating.

6. Exercise. Unfortunately, you can't just change what you eat, and expect to become super healthy. While it will have some amazing effects, exercise is a vital part of being healthy. That's why you should use a nutritious diet hand-in-hand with regular exercise.

# The China Study

One of the largest nutritional studies ever carried out, *The China Study*, surveyed more than 6,500 people. Over 65 different countries were included in the study. It confirmed that the power of plants really is strong, and there is no need to continue eating the meat and dairy rich diets that many westerners still have today.

# Sustainability

With the rate that the world's population is increasing, the amount of food that's required also grows. As there are more people on the planet, there needs to be a higher amount of food for everyone. In turn, that increases the amount of pressure that's being placed on nature, as well as global economies. Think about how much more space, water, nutrients from plants, and favorable weather is required to meet the rising demands for food. You can't avoid the fact that there is a finite amount of food that the environment can produce for the human race. The system for growing and manufacturing foods that is in place at the moment, simply cannot continue as it is. Eventually, the whole thing is going to fall apart, because it's just not sustainable.

Even though the animal agricultural industry makes up a huge amount of the world's market, it is extremely inefficient. Producing meat, dairy, and other animal goods, uses immense amounts of natural resources. About one quarter of the planet's land is completely dedicated to livestock that needs to graze. In addition to that, more than 30 percent of the land is used to grow feed for animals.

Water is another precious resource that needs to be taken care of. Around 70 percent of fresh water supplies are used for farming, but about a third of that is used for growing feed for food animals. All of the animals that are raised for the food industry produce almost 15 percent of the planet's greenhouse emissions, according to the United Nations Food and Agriculture Organization (FAO). However, some other organizations, such as the Worldwatch Institute, set that number closer to 50 percent.

Livestock needs to eat plenty of feed to stay strong and healthy (until it's time for the slaughterhouse). The sad fact is, all of the resources that are poured into growing feed, could simply be used to grow plants for people to eat in the first place. That would take a huge amount of strain of the ecosystem, as well as the world's economies. The land is degraded by livestock as well, which works to upset the natural ecosystem.

With just a little bit of information at your disposal, it's easy to see that eating vegan and vegetarian food isn't just good for your body — it's good for the entire planet's future. There are more people realizing just how destructive our modern agricultural industry is to Mother Nature. The key to leaving a better future to generations that will follow, lies in choosing sustainable sources of food, among other resources.

# Moral Reasons

Are you torn between your love of things like steak or bacon, and that nagging feeling in the back of your mind, when you eat them? It is highly likely that it's *guilt*, from causing the suffering and inevitable death of countless animals. There is no avoiding the fact that eating meat means contributing to their pain. Please don't kid yourself into thinking that you only eat animals that were "painlessly slaughtered", because there really is no such thing. It is not difficult to find images and video of what goes on in slaughter houses all over the world — and that includes first world countries. If you get that nagging feeling, the next time you're chowing down on a burger, it might be your good conscience trying to guide you.

The best case scenario for many food animals, if you can use the word "best", generally goes as follows: they are transported to a facility that is dedicated to slaughtering them. The animals in these slaughterhouses are able to hear and smell what is going on around them. Often, they are able to actually see their fellow creatures being killed. Anyone who believes that these animals are oblivious about what's going on, has never owned a pet before.

When animals struggle, which happens more than you would want to know, workers can become quite frustrated with them. Under strict deadlines, and trying to finish their workloads as quickly as possible, abuse does take place. If someone tells you that the slaughter of food animals is humane, they are delusional. There are plenty of resources out there where you can learn more about these industries in your area. This book will not go into too much detail. It's about the power of plants, and the positive things that they can do for your body — and that's a wholly positive thing.

# Vegetarian versus Vegan

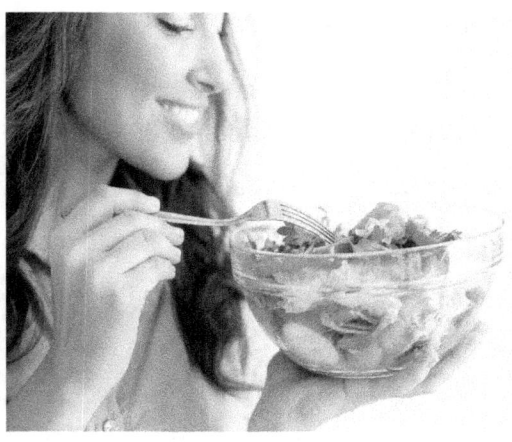

Jumping right into being a vegan can be too difficult for most people. It's often a good idea to turn vegetarian first, so that you can get used to a milder lifestyle change. This is a good step, and it's impressive it is own right. However, dairy products are some of the most fattening foods around. Think about the purpose of milk, and how that related to people. A cow produces milk to feed a calf, so that it can grow big, strong, and even fat. It is not intended for humans to drink. People don't continue to drink their mother's milk into later life, so why would they need to drink a cow's milk? In what way is consuming dairy natural? If you give it just a few minutes of thought, it's easy to see that society's views have become incredibly backwards.

## *What Do They Eat?*

In order to be a vegetarian, a person must not eat meat, including poultry and fish. If it was a living animal, you can safely assume that it's off the menu for vegetarians. However, they do eat other animal products, like dairy and eggs, which did not require any killing to be obtained. There are variations on this, like lacto-vegetarians, who eat dairy but not eggs. There are also ovo-vegetarians, who eat eggs but not dairy. Another type is pescetarianism, where people do eat seafood. Of course, this is not considered a true form of vegetarianism, by many people who don't eat any meat at all.

Vegans are more particular with what they do and don't eat. You can rule out anything that comes from an animal, including meat, poultry, fish, eggs, dairy, and even honey, which comes from bees. In addition to this, many vegans avoid purchasing products that are made from animals, including leather, fur, feather down, and cosmetics that have been tested on animals.

It should go without saying at this point in the book, that vegans *do* eat plenty of vegetables, fruits, grains and nuts.

Many people eat vegan diets due to allergies in animal products. These people are known as "dietary vegans", and it's not necessarily a choice that they have made. Others choose to turn vegan because of one, many, or all of the reasons listed previously in this book. Primarily, vegans believe that animals are not on this planet to be used as commodities, and exploited. This ties in with a strong respect for all living creatures, and certainly isn't something that should be mocked (as often happens, sadly).

# Going Plant-Based

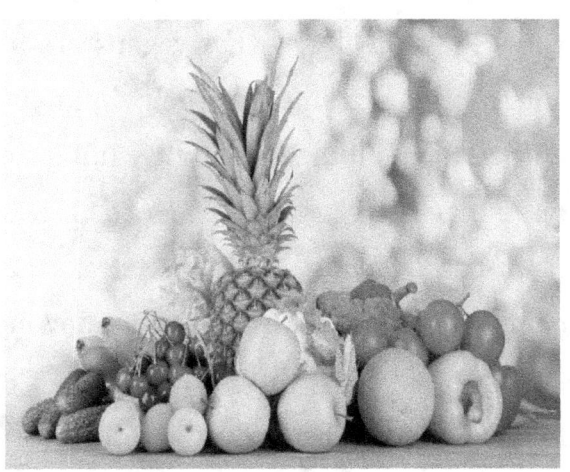

## *Quick Tips*

If you are reading this book, there's a pretty good chance that you're interested in becoming vegan. You might not be quite sure about whether or not you're ready to take that plunge. Simply mentioning the idea to your friends and family members might inspire a host of passionate responses. They will probably tell you that it's not natural, or it's too hard. People will say that vegans are all angry and extreme in their opinions. Forget about all that negativity, and focus on the positive aspects of switching to plant-based foods. Next, be clear that *going vegan isn't hard*. Avoid allowing anyone to tell you otherwise. The following tips will show you just how easy it can be:

## Do Your Research

No one is born knowing what they should eat to stay healthy. In fact, the evidence is all too clear that most people *don't* know how to eat a healthy diet, or they simply choose not to do so. You will need to have plenty of determination and a thirst for knowledge, if you're going to become a healthy vegan. It's still a pretty new thing, compared to other dietary lifestyles. You're going to need to be willing to research, ask questions, experiment, and of course *read food labels.* However, if you were not the type of person who asked questions, you might not be interested in changing your ways.

## Seek Help

Most vegans started out eating meat and other animal products. They decided to make the change at some point, and probably didn't have the slightest idea about how to do so. Don't be afraid to ask others for help. You're not alone, even if you don't know any vegans or vegetarians personally. The Internet is a brilliant resource, as you surely know. Join some online groups, and take part it discussions. If you're ever unsure about something, don't hesitate to ask people for help.

It's a good idea to ask your doctor for advice, and to give you a medical checkup. If you want to get yourself looked at after eating vegetarian or vegan food for some time, try keeping a food journal. This will make it easy to show your doctor exactly what you have been eating. If there's anything that you're not including in your diet, like enough vitamin B12 or protein, for example, they can let you know. Remember that doctors are not specialists in nutrition, so they're not guaranteed to have all the right answers about every type of diet.

**Take Things Slow**

The final goal is to remove animal products from your diet entirely. Let's assume that you are currently eating meat, dairy, eggs, etc. There are people who make the change to being vegan practically overnight, and that could be a good approach for you to take. However, if you need more time, don't worry. Like with other big lifestyle changes, it will probably take some time to get used to turning vegan. Everyone is also different, so there's no guaranteed method for change.

To begin with, making slight changes in your everyday eating routine is a good idea. If you tend to eat meat or dairy with almost every meal, try to reduce that to start with. Maybe you could take the ham or roast beef off your lunchtime sandwich, at least once a week. If you're comfortable with that, and still feeling motivated, you could remove the meat from all of your lunches. You could try to have just one day a week where you eat only vegan food, and gradually increase that to two days, then three, and so on.

If you have cow's milk with your coffee or cereal, try to swap to a plant-based alternative. There are loads to choose from, and many of them are quite tasty. Organic is best, and avoid cheap soy products, as they are often unhealthy. Almond or oat milk is a great choice, but why not mix things up?

**Don't Do Things by Half**
If you're going to make this change — do it properly. Avoid letting your body miss

out on everything it needs. Simply cutting animal products out of your diet will not automatically make you healthy. There are plenty of vegan junk foods around, and eating them all day is going to make you feel pretty lousy. Consume a good range of nutritious plant foods, with plenty of them being *whole* foods. Be sure that you get all of the vitamins, minerals, and nutrients that a healthy body requires. If this means taking supplements for now, until you can adapt to a more varied diet, that's perfectly fine. Lots of meat eaters take supplements as well, because it's often a more practical way to get everything you need.

## Keep Telling Yourself Why

No one decides to make these types of changes without their own good reasons.

What motivates you to stop eating meat, or animal products completely? Maybe you're just looking to cut down on those things, while increasing your plant intake. Whatever your reasons are for starting this change, always keep it at the forefront of your mind. You're going to have at least a few bad days, and probably realize that it's harder than you anticipated. Just breathe deeply, try to clear your mind, and think about the "why".

It can be hard to stay motivated if you are doing this on your own. If that's the case, read books about the subject, watching helpful and motivational videos, and write yourself little notes that you'll see regularly.

Have you decided to move away from

animal-based foods in order to help stop animal cruelty? That's wonderful, so how about reminding yourself just who you're helping? Visit a local animal shelter, or just go and be around some animals that are traditionally used for food. See for yourself how much personality each one of them has, and how many lives you are literally saving, just by changing your diet. This is a brilliant way to reaffirm exactly why you made this commitment in the first place.

**Keep Trying**

You are probably going to fall off the wagon at some point, especially when you're only just getting started. Don't think that you've failed miserably, simply because you caved in a ate some fried chicken, or a pepperoni pizza. Don't just throw it all away, and go back to your old ways, even if you do experience some small lapses in discipline. It *will* get easier, and you won't need to use will power in time. Eventually, saying "no" to meat and other animal products, will be easier than resisting the urge to drink poison (which should basically be the easiest thing you can think of!)

# Getting Started

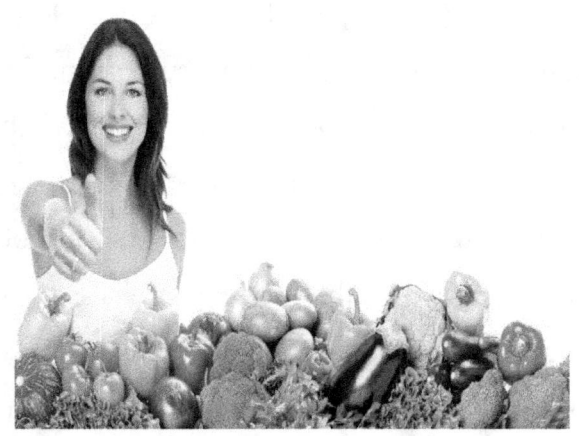

The quick tips listed previously will help you to get started, but the following advice is a little more specific. Let's assume that you have just decided to make the change to a plant-based diet, this very day. It's best to make small changes, and know when you're pushing yourself too hard.

***Cut Out Meat Slowly***

This step can be divided into several smaller stages, to make it easier to manage. As mentioned in the "Quick Tips" section, you can begin by having a meatless day per week (meat-free Mondays anyway?). Once you have successfully done that, and you're not having any trouble staying meatless on that one day, it's time to expand, but be sure that you really are ready. Another good idea is to remove red meat from your diet first, and then something else like poultry, etc. You can do this as slowly as you like. If you take a full month to move through each stage of your plan, that's totally fine. Heck, if you need even *more* time than a month, there's nothing stopping you. Just be sure to write down your plan, because it might be easy to forget over a long period of time.

As you remove meat from your diet, be sure that you're replacing it with other nutritionally equal foods. You're going to need other sources for things like protein, and probably iron. Ask your doctor, or another health care worker, if you need some more advice.

### Cut Out Eggs

Once you've stopped eating meat, you'll technically be a vegetarian. That means you're already halfway there, and many people are happy to remain at this step. However, since animal products are harmful, whether they're meat, dairy, or eggs — this book really aims to get people to convert entirely to being vegans. It might be easy to assume that eggs are cruelty free, and to think there's less reason to stop eating them. However, taking a look at where the hens who lay those eggs are kept, and the suffering they go through, should clear things up.

Once again, take this as slowly as you need to, and be sure that you're replacing those egg-based nutrients with suitable plant alternatives. Some people will tell you that eggs are required to properly prepare things like baked goods, burger patties, or pasta. That's not true, because there are common vegan alternatives.

### Cut Out Dairy

Is it so difficult for most people because they just love milk too much to give it up? There are *plenty* of tasty and varied alternatives out there, so this is not typically the case. Many people will tell you that they could just never give up eating *cheese*. This is where many of you might want to draw the line. There are a lot of great vegan alternatives on the market these days, but it can still be hard to give up things like pizza, or Parmesan cheese on your spaghetti.

This step might actually be more difficult than removing meat from your diet (it certainly was for yours truly). If it helps you, try to think of all of the great things that you *can* eat, instead of focusing on what you're missing out on.

### The World is yours!

Now that you've removed all animal based foods from your diet, it's time to celebrate. You can focus on eating healthier, whole foods that come from plants entirely. Not only will you feel a lot better for doing so, both physically and emotionally — but you'll be doing your part to reduce the strain that people put on the planet. If you don't believe this is true, just go back to the chapter about the benefits of going vegan, and read those points again.

# What Should You Eat?

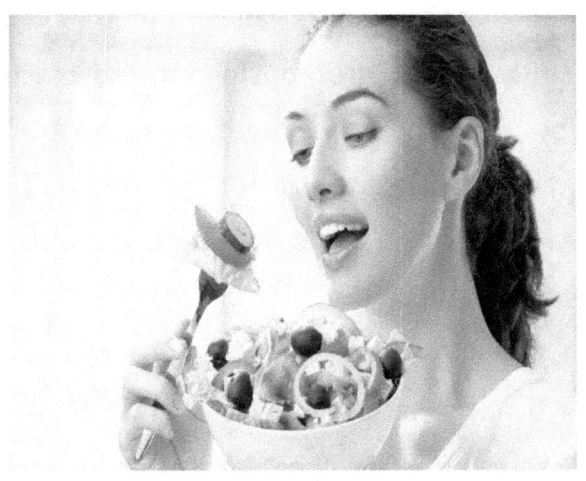

So, you have decided to eat more plants, or perhaps to switch to them entirely. It seems like a pretty simple concept, but many people are unsure what to do next, after making the decision. The best way to benefit from the power of plants, is to try and stick to a whole-food diet, based around plants. That means you should be trying to eat mostly foods that are not refined much. Cutting animal-based foods out of your diet might not do you much good, if you're going to be eating nothing but frozen dinners and canned soup. Those things are considered processed foods, but they're not always bad. It's best to read labels if you're not sure, and try to eat things that are as close to their natural state as possible.

A healthy, whole-food vegan diet is one that contains vegetables, fruits, whole grains, and legumes. You will naturally be excluding *all* meat (including fish and chicken), eggs, and dairy. Along with those things, it's a healthier choice to avoid overly refined foods, including sugars, flours, and oils that have gone through unwholesome processes. White sugar and bleached flour are a couple of examples.

This might all seem pretty overwhelming right now, especially if you have never learned much about nutrition and the way that food is manufactured and sold. Don't worry, because this will all be much easier to understand, in the near future. People have been eating whole foods since the beginning of known history. Once you get going, you'll probably start to *crave* all of the good things, which make up a complete and healthy vegan, or vegetarian, diet.

You don't need to miss out on any of your favorite meals either. You can use the following ingredients to create popular foods, including pasta, pizza, burritos, stews, burgers, BBQ foods, and so on. Anything that you can make with meat and animal products, you can make just as well without them. In fact, your plant-based alternatives will be *better*, since they'll be a lot healthier.

Here are the different types of foods that you should become familiar with, and some examples from each group:

### *Vegetables*

These include collard greens, lettuce, cauliflower, broccoli, Brussels sprouts, cucumber, spinach, squash, zucchini, eggplant, and kale.

### *Tubers*

These are also vegetables, yes, but it helps to place them in a separate category. Tubers include vegetables like yams, potatoes, sweet potatoes, carrots, beets, parsnips, radishes, and turnips.

### Fruit

This includes all of those natural, sweet treats, like grapes, berries, bananas, oranges, and apples.

### Whole grains

While not fruits or vegetables, these do come from plants, and will make up an important part of your new diet. These include rice, oats, whole wheat, barley, quinoa, buckwheat, amaranth, and millet.

### Legumes

You might also know these as "pulses". They are things like chickpeas, kidney beans, lima beans, black beans, cannellini beans, and lentils.

# Don't Focus on Single Nutrients

In modern culture, people tend to focus on single nutrients when they are buying or preparing meals. Just listen to the way that people call meats "proteins", instead of their proper names. It's a common view that people should eat meat for protein, fish for omega-3s, dairy for calcium, and plant foods for other various vitamins and minerals. You should leave that type of thinking behind right now. It's outdated and actually quite harmful to your health. Why do many people consume more meat and animal products than they need to? Protein is usually what people are after these days, especially if they're taking part in an exercise routine. Not only do people eat way more protein than they actually need, by doing this, but they eat a lot of other harmful substances to an extreme. These include things like bad cholesterol and saturated fats.

Foods are not make up of single nutrients, so it does little good to think of them that way. Just about any food that you can think of has *many* different nutrients. There are so many that it would be practically impossible to keep track of them from day to day. A diet of whole, plant-based ingredients, will contain *everything* that you need, as part of a large package. There is only the single exception of vitamin B12, which can no longer be absorbed from vegan foods, due to the way in which they are farmed these days. Don't worry, because a cheap and simple supplement is all that's required.

## More than Just Vegetables

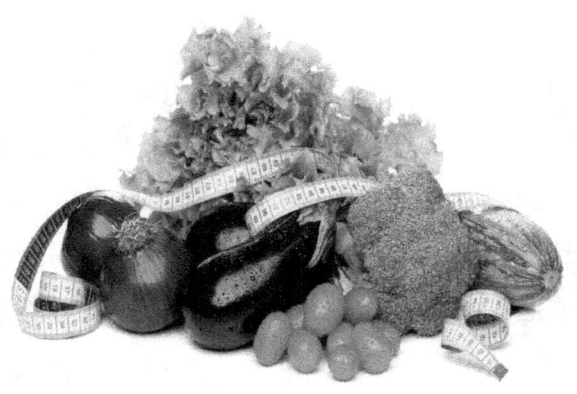

People like to think of vegans and vegetarians as people who just eat green salads for every meal. Maybe that helps them to feel superior, while they're ruining their health, the planet, and causing endless suffering, all to get another steak. Yes, things like spinach and other greens *do* make up a majority of plant-based diets. However, there is much more to it than that, as you have probably guessed after looking at the different food groups listed above.

Leafy greens are an essential part of a natural, plant-based lifestyle. However, you would need to eat *a lot* of them in order to get your daily nutritional needs. It just wouldn't be practical, or even possible. In fact, a lot of people probably fail at turning vegan or vegetarian, because they attempt to eat nothing but typical salad foods. You might wonder why you should bother to eat them at all, since they can't give your body what it needs. They contain a lot of great things, which are essential for staying healthy.

No matter how good your intentions are, or how much you manage to eat, a person simply can't live off these types of vegetables alone. Eventually, your body would start to become starved, since it wouldn't be getting enough daily calories. If you know anyone who tried to switch to a plant-based diet, but failed miserably, there's a good chance they were just doing it completely wrong. This might be the cause of the popular opinion, that vegans don't get enough necessary calories.

If you can't just eat salad vegetables for survival, what *do* you need to include in your diet?

In the United States, as well as many other western and developed countries, people are used to planning their meals around what type of meat they will eat. This is obviously going to be different for you, should you choose to continue a plant-based eating plan. However, the main stars of your plate will now be those delicious, starchy foods that many people also love. These types of things have been given a bad name, and are commonly viewed as not being healthy. Think of things like potatoes or sweet potatoes, peas and corn, whole rice or buckwheat, and beans and lentils. These are going to be a primary part of your new diet. The ways that these things are prepared will be different than you're probably used to. Instead of mixing them with dairy or saturated oils, they'll be prepared in different ways.

# Essential Vegan Items

Along with all of the usual pantry items that most people buy, there are some special extras that are a must for vegans and vegetarians alike. However, these things are also recommended for those looking to eat less meat, which is the very goal of this book. In order to get all of the nutrition, flavor, and texture that is required for healthy, fulfilling meals, consider stocking your kitchen with the following items.

## Legumes

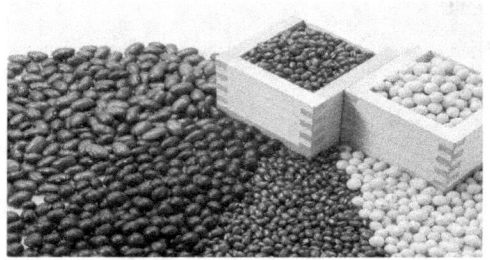

It's good to make sure that you have lots of different beans and other legumes. You can buy them dried or canned (look for BPA free cans), so why not buy a selection of each type? Chickpeas and lentils are two of the most popular types with vegans and vegetarians, and they can go into just about any dish you care to make. The canned variety are more convenient, since they don't need to be re-hydrated, and are quick to cook. Dried lentils are also pretty easy to prepare, and take little cooking time.

## Oats

Oatmeal is a quick and high-energy breakfast that can also help to lower your cholesterol. Why not keep a bag of pressed oats handy at all times, so you never have to go without a hearty meal at the start of the day. They are also a delight to bake with, and can be readily added to cakes and cookies, to name just a couple of things.

## Nuts

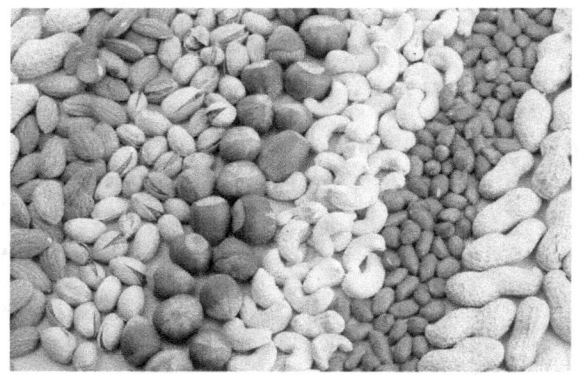

Forget what people say about nuts containing too much fat. They contain *good* fats, which are required by the human boyd. In fact, you can let yourself go totally *nuts* about eating nuts! They're good to eat by themselves as snacks, in cooking, or as salad ingredients. You can even grind them up, and add them to dishes, without affecting the texture too much.

## Dried Fruit

Make sure that you don't buy the brands that come covered in syrup or sugar. Like nuts, these are also great to eat by themselves, or to use in deserts and even savory meals. They keep for ages, if stored in sealed containers, so you can always have them on hand.

## Grains

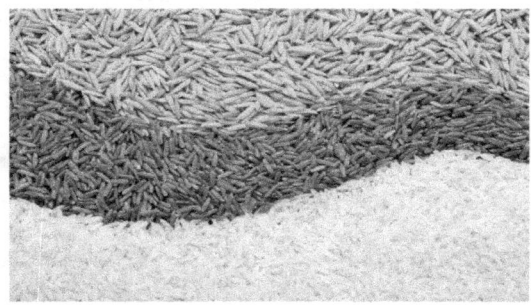

Since these are typically dried, you can stock up on plenty, and they will keep for a long time. Rice is extremely cheap, and brown rice is super nutritious. There are other types like spelt, quinoa, and millet too. Don't limit yourself to just eating white rice with your meals, because you won't be getting a very varied selection of grains.

## Tempeh

You might not have heard of this one before, but it's pretty common. It does need to be kept in the fridge. However, you can use it as a regular source of protein, and it can even be frozen.

## Tofu

Here's another item that you will need to keep in the fridge, or the freezer. It comes in a range of different textures, and you can buy it already flavored. Just be sure to check that there aren't to many salts, sugars, or other nasty additives in the flavoring.

## Veggie Stock

You can purchase this, and it's an extremely convenient way to add a flavor base to dishes. However, making it from scratch is not only cheaper and usually healthier, but it's very satisfying to eat something you created with your own two hands. When you're buying vegetable stock, be sure to get a brand that doesn't load it up with chemicals and salt.

## Miso

Miso paste comes in both light and dark varieties. It's an easy way to add a lot of depth of flavor to meals. You can even use to make a simple broth, to enjoy for supper on those cold winter nights.

## Nutritional Yeast

This isn't something that most people would even think about buying. If you want to create a "cheesy" type of sauce or food coating, this is an essential ingredient. There are also different types that have added nutritional value, such as vitamin B12.

## Maple Syrup

If you're going vegan, it's time to say goodbye to honey. That's an animal product, so it's big no-no. Maple syrup is perfectly fine, however, and it goes well with all sorts of foods (pancakes, anyone?).

## Olive Oil

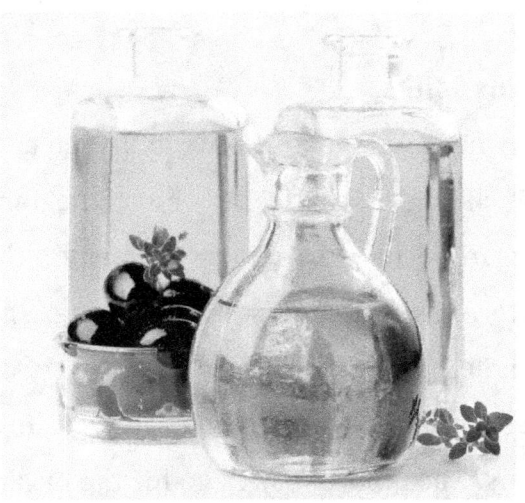

Cold pressed, extra virgin olive oil contains the most nutritional value. It also tastes amazing on just about anything that you want to make. You can use any oil that contains primarily unsaturated fats, but this one has been a mainstay all over the world, for centuries. It's great for adding to salad dressing, or putting right on top of meals, like pasta. While you can cook with it, be mindful of the relatively low heat point.

## Faux-Milks

Saying goodbye to cow's milk isn't too much of a hassle for most beginner vegans. There are just so many other alternatives that it's like opening up a whole new world. There is soy, rice, oat, cashew, macadamia, and almond milk, plus much more. Try to go for the organic brands if you can, and take a look at the added ingredients as well. You'd be surprised by how many cheaper brands are loaded with preservatives and sugar, especially with long-life milks.

## Pickled and Preserved Vegetables

You might not always feel like cooking up some veggies. When the urge to snack comes along, it's better to reach for a jar of vegetables, instead of chowing down on sweets or potato chips. If you buy products that are fermented, you will be giving your body some good bacteria. These can help to keep your intestinal system in good order.

## Soy Sauce

This is a long-loved staple for vegetarians and vegans. It can add a hit of savory flavor to practically any dish, or be enjoyed as a topping for things like rice and lentils.

## Fruits

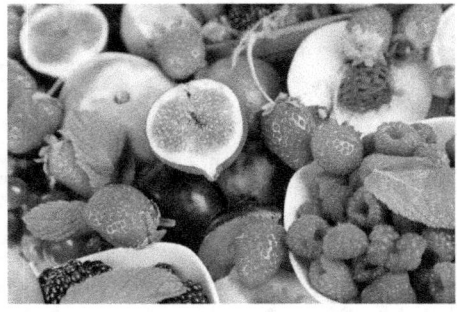

They can be tasty, sweet treats by

themselves, used in your favorite desserts, or even in savory meals. Here are some of the more popular and nutritious types that you can try:

Apricot

Apple

Berries

Banana

Cranberries

Cantaloupe

Figs

Grapes

Grapefruit

Kiwi fruit

Limes

Lemons

Melons

Oranges

Pineapple

Pears

Papaya

Prune

Plum

Raisins

## Vegetables

There are a lot of them out there, so here is a thorough list of many things that you should consider trying:

Avocado

Asparagus

Bell peppers

Beets

Brussels sprouts

Broccoli

Cabbage

Celery

Cauliflower

Cucumber

Carrots

Collard greens

Eggplant

Green peas

Green beans

Garlic

Kale

Leeks

Mustard Greens

Mushrooms

Mushrooms

Onions

Olives

Potato

Parsley

Seaweed

Spinach

Sweet potato

Swiss chard

Squash

Tomatoes

Turnips

Yams

# Don't Want to Quit Meat?

Many people are probably reading this book in an attempt to become healthier, but have no desire to actually quit eating animal products. Can you have the "best" of both worlds? Yes, you can! It's certainly possible to keep eating the things that you enjoy, or that you feel are important for your own diet, while introducing more plant-based foods into your daily meals.

Just take some advice from vegans, and the ways that they use plants to sustain life and wellness. Even if you think that "vegan" is somewhat of a dirty word, and would never be caught dead giving up meat, cheese, eggs, etc. — you can still benefit from this book. Take a smarter approach to what you put in your grocery shopping cart each week, and give some thought to what you're actually eating.

Below are the vegan habits that everyone should consider adopting:

## Add More Vegetables

You don't have to be a vegetarian or vegan to benefit from this wonderful tip. If you take just one thing away from this entire book — it should be to eat a lot more vegetables, every singe to day. It doesn't matter if you make a pizza that's covered with ham and pepperoni. You can still add things like mushrooms, capsicum, eggplant, zucchini, and so on. Never assume that you can only have one or the other, or that eating meat somehow negates the positive effects of plants.

Naturally, you're not going to need to eat the same types of vegetables, unless you're going totally vegan. Pile on more of the non-starchy veggies, as well as lots of greens. They contain loads of things that you cannot get from meat and animal products. You will be injecting your body with healthier protein, vitamins, minerals, that all-important fiber, and antioxidants, among other things.

Make a decision right now, to add at least a couple of additional vegetables to everything meal that you make. Never again be satisfied with just meat and white grains, and you will soon start to realize how great vegan food can make you feel.

## Use More Herbs and Spices

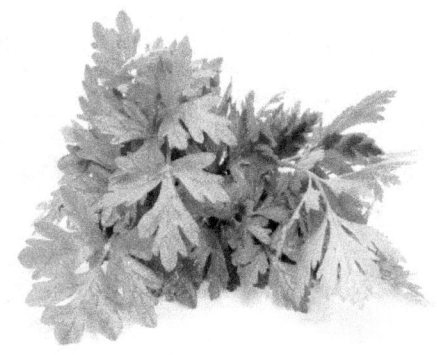

If you're used to flavoring everything with butter and salt, it might seem a little hard to cook with herbs spices. For those who never use those things, having a well-rounded spice rack quickly becomes an essential. All of the best chefs in the world use herbs and spices anyway, no matter what type of food they're cooking. Not only do they make food taste *better*, but they bring along plenty of nutritional value. By mixing up the different types that you add to your other ingredients, you can create many different meals, using the same things.

## Opt for Plant-Based Protein

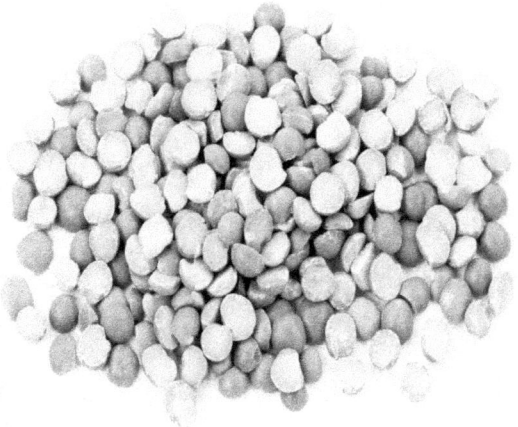

Rather than trying to meet all of your daily protein requirements by eating meat, how about increasing the plant-based protein that you consume? Legumes are a key part of the vegan diet. They're loaded with protein and fiber, but also have tons of minerals, vitamins, and other nutritious components. As mentioned earlier in this book, they are also free from that harmful animal protein that can contribute to a range of medical problems, like heart disease and cancer. Don't let people tell you that they're unhealthy, due to high amounts of carbohydrates. Lentils, beans, and chickpeas are wonderfully nutritious, and the human body does need a certain amount of good, complex carbs each day as well as protein.

If you're game to try something that's probably a little unusual for many people — how about tempeh or tofu? These are staples for many vegans and vegetarians, and they can go well in just about any dish you want to use them in.

## Ditch the Mayo

Do you love putting mayonnaise on your sandwiches? No one can blame you, because it's pretty tasty to most people. However, it's made mostly out of egg yolks, so vegans don't eat it. Does that mean your next lunchtime meal is going to be dry and flavorless? Certainly not! By removing that calorie-rich, egg-filled spread, and choosing a healthier option — you can do wonders for your health.

This is good advice, even if you just want a healthier choice of vegan sauces, like most ketchups and BBQ sauces. You can even get creative, and try something like mashed avocado, or homemade hummus.

## Cook Your Own Meals

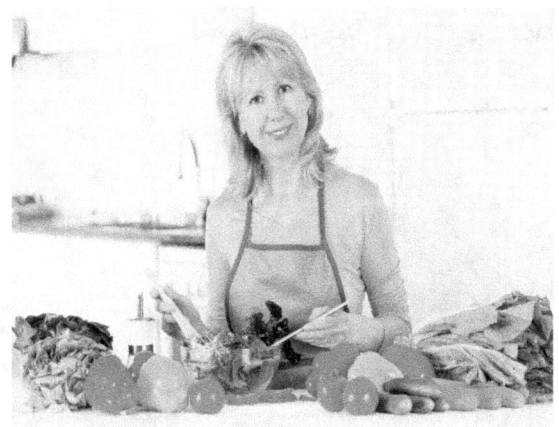

When you can't just grab any old things off the supermarket shelf, it almost becomes a necessity to makes things from scratch. This is something that everyone can benefit from. Not only does it teach people to be more conscious of what's going into their mouths, but it gives better results, and healthier meals. Spending some extra time cooking in the kitchen, can become a fun and fulfilling hobby. It is also a good way to save money that would have otherwise gone toward buying pre-

leahciM K

packaged food items.

# CONCLUSION

So, have you been sold on the miracle that is a plant-based diet? I certainly hope so, but many people are probably still skeptical. It can take a lot to convince a person to change the very food that they regularly eat. Generally, people are raised as omnivores, eating food from animals and plants alike. You might believe that there just isn't anything wrong with do so, and that's absolutely fine.

The main goal in writing this book has been to try and get people thinking more about the ways that the foods they eat, affect their overall health. Not only that, but the ways that our food impacts the planet, as well as the other living creatures on it.

If you have taken very little away from this book, hopefully it has at least convinced you to start eating more plant-based foods. You don't have to make big changes, and you can still start to see some great benefits. Introducing just a few more serves of vegetables, fruits, and whole grains into your diet every day, can do wonders.

Please, do give it a try, and remember all of the great health benefits that you can expect in time. But be aware that it *will* take *time*, and you might not notice huge changes. It would take a larger shift in diet to notice anything too major. And no one can logically expect things to happen overnight.

Thank you for taking the time to learn

more about the power of plants, and why you should eat more. I wish you all the best health in the future.

www.ingramcontent.com/pod-product-compliance
Lightning Source LLC
Chambersburg PA
CBHW071212280526
45787CB00002B/651